The Essential Oils Quick Guide: On a Budget

Ashley Quiroz

ISBN-13:978-1717023582
ISBN-10:1717023584

DEDICATION

To mom's like me, who want quality at a great price!

CONTENTS

EVERYDAY
ESSENTIAL OILS
UNDER $21
AND
HOW TO LIVE OFF REWARD
PROGRAMS

WHAT ARE ESSENTIAL OILS?

Essential oils are the regenerating, oxygenating, and immune defense properties of plants. Essential oils are so small in molecular size that they can quickly penetrate the skin and cell walls. In fact, essential oils can affect every cell of the body within 20 minutes and then be metabolized like other nutrients. We share a majority of our DNA with plants, so our bodies easily utilize those benefits! Essential oils promote emotional, physical, and spiritual health. There is no standard for essential oils set by any government agency in North America. So labeling fraud is rampant. To be sure you are getting therapeutic grade oils, you need to know your grower, distiller, packager and distributor because anywhere along this chain of delivery, oils can be compromised. There is a difference in quality.

Applying Essential Oils

Aromatically: You can smell them from the bottle, your hands, or an essential oil diffuser. They have profound emotional impact, as well as various physical benefits. Essential oils can boost your mood and freshen the air. They also stimulate the brain, help bring balance and are oxygenating.

Topically: Apply to areas of concern for example your neck, bottoms of feet, or pulse points. Be sure to dilute with a fatty carrier oil for sensitive skin or with hot, spicy oils like oregano, cinnamon, and lemongrass. You can add them to bath salts & lotions for DIY body care. Add to water to make a room spray or even blend together to make your own Roll-Ons.

Internally: Many oils are labeled for internal consumption, many oils that can be found in grocery stores are labeled "Do Not Ingest". Make sure they are safe for internal use before ingesting. Drink citrus or peppermint in water in glass, stainless steel, or ceramic only. Put a drop on or under your tongue, gargle with water, or rub into the roof of your mouth Put drops in an empty vegetable capsule and dilute, if desired.

Applying Essential Oils to Children 2 Years and Up

Aromatically: Smell them from the bottle, depending how coordinated your child is, a drop in the palm and inhale. Diffusing works great for children!

Topically: Apply to areas of concern, neck, bottoms of feet, or pulse points. Dilute with a fatty carrier oil for sensitive skin. With hot, spicy oils oregano, cinnamon, and lemongrass dilute 20 parts EO/80 parts carrier oil and apply to feet.

Internally: Mothers have given their children essential oils internally and have had success. The book, *Gentle Babies* by Debra Raybern, is a great book for more info on how to safely use oils on babies, children and pregnant mommas.

Disclaimer

I am a mom who uses essential oils for my family, I am not a doctor or a medical provider. These are things that I have done to care for my own family. Please consult with your doctor about any health concerns you may have. I recommend you do some research and make an informed decision that you are comfortable with.

Less really is more

Essential oils are highly concentrated plant extracts. A little goes a long way! That being said, don't be fooled, If you get your oils from a legit and honest company, a small 5- or 10-ml bottle is very potent and will likely be enough to last you many months with frequent use. The Idea of " if a little is good, a lot is better" is not always correct. Start low and go slow. In most cases 1-2 drops are adequate and using more may waste product. Depending on the EO you can gradually build up to 3-4 uses per day if desired.

Essential Oils Reference Guide

There are many powerful essential oils. To find out everything about them I suggest an Essential Oils Reference Guide. You can find them online at Life Science Publishing. This little book is just a quick guide for us on a budget.

<u>**Addiction Recovery Support:**</u>

Note: I only know what helped for me, go with an oil that is most like your addiction. If it is an upper go with oils that uplift you. If it is a downer, then go with the ones that bring calming. Always have some form of support group if you are struggling with recovering from addiction, this is a tough battle to go through, don't go it alone! Also, don't hesitate to consult with a trained professional.

Single: Black Pepper, Cedarwood, Clove, Fennel, Lemongrass, Orange, Peppermint, Tangerine, Wintergreen

For Adults: One drop in hand, inhale deeply and exhale any of these oils. In this case you are looking for immediate relief and changing the way your brain reacts to stimulation. Inhaling and meditation is the best method for this.

For Children: Any oils above, diluted 50/50, on bottom of feet, massage into neck/back area. Also, you can diffuse any of the oils listed in your child's room.

<u>**Inner Defense:**</u>

Singles: Clove, Lemon, Oregano, Spearmint, Tangerine, Eucalyptus Blue

For Adults: One drop in hand, inhale deeply and exhale

any of these oils. Clove, Lemon, Oregano, Spearmint and Tangerine can be found as vitality oils and work great ingested. Diffuse any of these oils in a diffuser. It works best when you are able to relax close by.

For Children: Any oils above, diluted 50/50, on bottom of feet. Oregano is a hot oil use on bottoms of feet and diluted 20/80. Diffuse any oils in child's room.

Bone, Joint, and Muscle Support:

Singles: Basil, Black Pepper, Clove, Eucalyptus Globulus, Ginger, Lemongrass, Marjoram, Nutmeg, Peppermint, Pine, Rosemary, Wintergreen

For Adults: Local and topical use recommended for relief of any discomforts. For preventative use: Basil, Black Pepper, Clove, Ginger, and Lemongrass are all great oils for internal consumption and can be found as a vitality oil.

For Children: Any oils above, diluted 50/50, on bottom of feet. My go to is wintergreen and clove diluted with coconut oil, apply on site.

Breast Feeding: Increasing Milk Supply

Singles: Celery Seed, Fennel, Basil

Use any of these with a carrier oil on breast (not nipple) after feeding to encourage milk flow. Fennel Vitality in a tsp of honey also works great.

<u>**Digestive Support:**</u>

Singles: Black Pepper, Celery Seed, Citronella, Clove, Dill, Eucalyptus Radiata, Fennel, Ginger, Grapefruit, Lemongrass, Marjoram, Peppermint, Spearmint, Tangerine

For Adults: Any oils above, diluted directly on stomach area. Any vitality oils under the tongue and lots of water.

For Children: Any oils above, diluted 50/50, directly on stomach or on bottom of feet. You can diffuse any of these in a child's room.

<u>**Emotional and Spiritual Support:**</u>

Singles: Bergamot, Lavender, Lemon, Orange, Pine, Sage, Cedarwood, Citronella, Fennel, Spearmint, Tangerine

For Adults: One drop in hand, inhale deeply and exhale any of these oils (the whole breathe and count to 10 concept).

For Children: Any oils above, diluted 50/50, on bottom of feet or into the back/area. You can diffuse any of these in a child's room.

Fortifying and Maintaining Body Systems

Singles: Black Pepper, Dill, Grapefruit, Lemon, Peppermint, Nutmeg, Rosemary.

For Adults: All the oils above can be found as a vitality oil and taken internally in water, honey, or vegetable capsule.

 For Children: Any oils above, diluted 50/50, on bottom of feet. You can diffuse any of these in a child's room.

Immune System Support

Singles: Basil, Clove, Cypress, Eucalyptus Blue, Eucalyptus Globulus, Eucalyptus Radiata, Lemon, Lemongrass, Oregano, Rosemary, Sage, Thyme

For Adults: One drop in hand, inhale deeply and exhale any of these oils. Make a roller bottle with equal amounts of each: Oregano, Clove, Basil, Thyme, Sage, and Lemon then top it off with a carrier oil and roll on your feet everyday.

For Children: Any oils above, diluted 50/50, on bottom of feet. Oregano is a hot oil, use on bottoms of feet and diluted 20/80 (or 10/90). Diffuse any oils in child's room. Diffuse at bath time along with a steamed bath or shower.

<u>Memory, Lack of Clarity, Brain fog</u>

Singles: Black Pepper, Lavender, Peppermint, Rosemary, Lemon, Orange

For Adults: One drop in hand, inhale deeply and exhale any of these oils. Kind of like a meditation concept. Breathe in and out to clear your mind and focus on your mission.

For Children: Any oils above, diluted 50/50, on bottom of feet. You can diffuse any of these in a child's room or school work area.

<u>Migraine Relief & Brain Support</u>

Singles: Basil, Clove, Eucalyptus Globulus, Eucalyptus Blue, Lavender, Marjoram, Peppermint, Rosemary, Spearmint, Wintergreen

For Adults: One drop in hand, inhale deeply and exhale any of these oils. Put one drop of peppermint and one drop of clove into palm, dip your thumb into the oil and then place onto the roof of your mouth. This opens the cranial sutures and stimulates the pineal gland and sends the beneficial molecules of the oils directly into the blood stream in your brain.

For Children: Any oils above, diluted 50/50, on bottom of feet or into the back/neck area. You can diffuse any of these in a child's room.

Oral Care

Singles: Clove, Wintergreen, Peppermint, Lemon, Oregano, Thyme

For Adults: Gargle or brush teeth with any of these oils with peroxide and baking soda. For direct relief put clove diluted with coconut oil on site.

For Children: 2 years+: One drop of clove into a small cup of peroxide and gargle. Or rub a diluted 50/50 mixture of coconut oil, clove and lemon directly onto gums for direct relief.

Metabolism Support

Note: What we eat and what we put on our bodies and what we are inhaling everyday plays a huge part in our health. GMO's, pesticides, laundry detergent, dryer sheets, household cleaners, lotions, make-up, shampoos, conditioners, perfume etc. can all have hormone disrupting chemicals which attribute to thyroid problems and metabolism issues that keep us over weight and fatigued. The good news is that there are lots of options for switching out the toxins for really good quality and great smelling alternatives.

Singles: Black Pepper, Fennel, Ginger, Grapefruit, Lemon, Lime, Nutmeg, Spearmint

For Adults: You can find clear vegetable capsules online or at health food stores. I like to make my own capsule with one drop grapefruit, ginger and black pepper and then filled with coconut or almond oil.

For Children: Any oils above, diluted 50/50, on bottom of feet. You can diffuse any of these in a child's room.

Respiratory and Throat/Sinus Support

Singles: Basil, Citronella, Eucalyptus Globulus, Peppermint, Eucalyptus Radiata, Eucalyptus Blue, Goldenrod, Cedarwood, Cypress, Lemongrass, Pine (Caution: Beware of pine essential oils mixed with turpentine, a low-cost filler that is potentially hazardous and even fatal.)

For Adults: One drop in hand, inhale deeply and exhale any of these oils. A roller bottle with equal amounts of each oil: Oregano, Clove, Basil, Thyme, Sage, and Lemon (can top off with a carrier oil) and roll on your feet every day. 50/50 Oregano and carrier oil in capsule. A "Eucalyptus Vapor Rub" recipe can be found online.

For Children: Any oils above, diluted 50/50, on bottom of feet. You can diffuse any of these in a child's room. Heavily dilute any combination of these in a carrier oil and rub on chest or back for a vapor rub.

Seasonal Changes: Immune Support

Singles: Fennel, Eucalyptus Blue, Lavender, Peppermint

For Adults: One drop in hand, inhale deeply and exhale any of these oils. Any Vitality oil, listed above, under the tongue or in a Vegetable Capsule. Lavender, Lemon, Peppermint is a good combo to blend and take internally.

For Children: Any oils above, diluted 50/50, on bottom of feet. You can diffuse any of these in a child's room. Make real lemonade with (local) honey for sweetness, add one drop Lavender, Lemon, Peppermint. Store in glass container with a tight seal. Drink during the day. Perfect for "on the go" outings to the park, zoo, etc.

Skin Care: Beauty

Note: After applying essential oils on the skin, use a natural skin cream to sooth the natural drying effect of some oils. As an aging woman, I don't mind spending a little more money on beauty and health.

Singles: Black Pepper, Lavender, Thyme, (the following are photosensitizing and should be used at night, when used during the day, avoid sunlight for 30 minutes) Tangerine, Orange, Lemon (also helps smooth blemishes) Lime, Grapefruit

Skin: Caring for Bruises

Singles: Clove, Lemongrass, Wintergreen, Peppermint

For All: Apply on Site. Clove, Wintergreen and Peppermint are hot oils, dilution is recommended.

Skin: Caring for Abscesses, Boils & Pimples

Single: Lavender, Oregano, Clove, Rosemary, Thyme

For Adults: Lavender (is good enough for day to day blemishes), Oregano (diluted 20/80) for more intense care.

For Children: Lavender, Oregano is a hot oil, use on dilute 20/80 (or 10/90) Apply on site. Use a toothpick to keep the oregano directly on site and off the skin.

Skin: Caring for Blisters

Singles: Lavender

For Adults and For Children: Lavender is my go to for all topical skin care on children's skin.

Skin: Caring for Insect Bites

Note: Essential oils can bring comfort to an insect bite, however, take bites seriously and find out what type of bite it is. Seek medical attention immediately if you suspect it is poisonous and/or fatal.

Singles: Basil, Lavender, Citronella, Eucalyptus Globulus, Grapefruit, Lime, Peppermint, Rosemary, Clove, Thyme

For Adults and Children: Apply any of these oils topically on site. Create a 15ml roller bottle blend of 20 drops clove and 20 drops grapefruit and top off with coconut oil for an "on the go" blend.

Skin: Caring for Small Open Wounds & Burns

Singles: Lavender

For Adults and For Children: Lavender (topically on area, for children dilute with coconut oil for even more care and support).

P.S We all know our children have emotions that come with bumps and bruises. Comfort them with your love along with essential oils for emotional support!

Stress & Hyperactivity Relief

Singles: Cedarwood, Dill, Fennel, Lavender, Lemon, Lime, Orange, Rosemary

For Adults: One drop in hand, inhale deeply and exhale any of these oils. Rub into back of neck or temple area. Kind of like a meditation concept. Breathe in and out, clear your mind and focus on your mission.

For Children: Any oils above, diluted 50/50, on bottom of feet, on back of neck or temple area. You can diffuse any of these in a child's room.

<u>**Urinary Tract & Bladder Support:**</u>

Singles: Oregano, Lemon, Lemongrass, Thyme, Rosemary, Clove

For Adults: Any of these oils can be found as vitality and can be put into capsule form. Remember, you only need one or two drops and always use more carrier oil than the essential oil. You can also add any to honey or into a glass (not plastic) of water and ingest that way.

For Children: Make some real lemonade and add lemon and honey for them to drink. Put a drop of lemon, lemongrass or grapefruit in a tsp of honey and have them ingest it. Drink lots of water.

Reward Programs

Auto Ship programs have a lot of Rewards. First, it saves me a trip to multiple stores, which was always so stressful with children. Also, it has been a bridge to exchange toxic cleaning and hygiene supplies, vitamins and now even my makeup for a natural non- toxic option. So let me tell you about it. You can customize your monthly order and save money. Choose your products and when your order processes. Change you order or cancel at any time. Receive reduced shipping rates and priority shipments of your favorite products. Gain access to exclusive monthly promotions. Discounted pricing on exclusive product kits. Reward Points with every order works like cash to use toward future orders. The longer you are on the auto ship plan the more you get back, so something like this, 1-3 months: 10 percent, 4-24 months: 20 percent and 25+ months: 25 percent of each order back in points. Also you get access to exclusive bonuses. In this case loyalty pays.

Let's talk about how to live off rewards. I order our vitamins every month on auto ship. I add my makeup and hygiene supplies to auto ship when they are running low. I only use quick order in an emergency. By the time I am running out of oils, I would have accumulated enough points back in cash to buy the oils I need. Getting my oils free by transferring my spending to a trusted company is priceless. This is a triple jackpot. I get quality vitamins for my family! I get my products mailed straight to my door and the company pays me back in reward points, then I buy my oils for free. Wait! There is more. Since I do spend over $190 a month (that I would have been spending somewhere else regardless) they send me free promotional items that keep my essential oil product collection growing with new products.

If you are ready to save time and money with the auto ship program speak to the person who signed you up or contact customer service, they will be glad to assist you.

<u>**Essential Oil Singles 5ml**</u>

EUCALYPTUS BLUE $15.50

GOLDENROD $15.75

BASIL $10.75

BERGAMOT $13.50

BLACK PEPPER $19.25

CELERY SEED $11.75

DILL $16.25

CLOVE $7.50

FENNEL $9.00

GINGER $13.50

JADE LEMON $11.00

LAVENDER $12.00

MARJORAM $14.75

NUTMEG $13.25

ORANGE $6.00

OREGANO $12.00

PEPPERMINT $10.25

ROSEMARY $7.75

SAGE $12.75

SPEARMINT $11.00

TANGERINE $7.75

THYME $14.50

<u>Essential Oil Singles 15ml</u>

CEDARWOOD $11.50

CITRONELLA $20.00

CLOVE $15.75

CYPRESS $19.75

EUCALYPTUS RADIATA $19.00

EUCALYPTUS GLOBULUS $14.75

FENNEL $17.75

GRAPEFRUIT $17.25

LEMON $11.50

LEMONGRASS $11.50

LIME $12.50

ORANGE $11.00

PINE $15.50

ROSEMARY $16.00

TANGERINE $16.50

WINTERGREEN $18.25

www.ingramcontent.com/pod-product-compliance
Lightning Source LLC
Chambersburg PA
CBHW061327250726
48657CB00003B/1084